Medical Disclaimer

You understand and acknowledge that readers of this
document are responsible for their own medical care,
treatment, and oversight. All content found in this
document, including: text, images, audio, or other
formats were created for informational purposes only.
The Content is not intended to be a substitute for
professional medical advice, diagnosis, or treatment.
Always seek the advice of your physician or other
qualified health provider with any questions you may
have regarding a medical condition. Never disregard
professional medical advice or delay in seeking it
because of something you have read in this document.

Medical information changes constantly. Therefore the
information in this document should not be
considered current, complete or exhaustive, nor
should you rely on such information to recommend a
course of treatment for you or any other individual.

If you think you may have a medical emergency, call your doctor, go to the emergency department, or call 911 immediately. We do not recommend or endorse any specific tests, physicians, products, procedures, opinions, or other information that may be mentioned in this document. Reliance on any information provided in this document is solely at your own risk.

Table of Contents

An Introductory to Red Light Therapy

Red Light Therapy is a treatment that could be helpful to your skin, muscle tissue, and different parts of your body to heal. Red Light Therapy works by exposing the affected area of your body to a lamp, device, or laser that has a distinctive red light. Red Light Therapy can also be called low-level laser therapy (LLLT), low-power laser therapy (LPLT), or photobiomodulation (PBM). The FDA has to approve the devices. Therefore the treatment is FDA approved.

How does Red Lamp Therapy Work?

The devices will deliver concentrated wavelengths of natural light into your skin. This is done with a small amount of heat that is not strong enough to burn you and does not hurt. It works by stimulating the parts of the cells that are called mitochondria, which are sometimes called "power generators." They absorb the treatment and then generate energy. Scientists speculate that this helps the cells fix themselves and tends to make them healthier. It helps stimulate healing in the skin and muscle tissue that has damage.

The treatments will help energize the production of elastin, fibroblasts, and collagen so that your skin will not sag or droop. Red lamp therapy increases circulation that will bring more nutrients and oxygen to your cells and tissues.

What Does it Treat and How Long Does it Take?

• Dementia

After 12 weeks of regular near-infrared light therapy on the head, and through the nose, you can get some results. Your memory will be improved, and so will your sleep. You will be less angry too.

• Androgenetic Alopecia

This disease causes you to lose your hair, and it does not grow back. You will use an in-home Red lamp therapy device. You will be able to grow thicker hair after 24 weeks.

• Dental Pain

Temporomandibular Dysfunction Syndrome is where you have pain, clicking, and tenderness in the jaw. After having Red lamp therapy, you find that you will have fewer symptoms. It would help if you started getting relief from the pain in less than 20 minutes.

• Osteoarthritis

This is where the cartilage that cushions the ends of your bones wears down as time goes on. It can harm any joint in the body. The most common areas that are affected are the knees, hips, spine, and hands. The pain can be lessened in under 20 minutes of near-infrared light therapy.

• Tendinitis

The thick fibrous cords that attach the muscle to the bone are the tendons. Tendinitis is when that tendon is inflamed or irritated. This will cause you pain and tenderness on the outside of the joint. This is commonly seen in the shoulders, elbows, wrists, knees, and heels.

• Wrinkles

A typical stage of aging is when you get wrinkles. A major cause of wrinkles is sun exposure. Two other things that cause wrinkles are smoking and pollutants around you.

• Skin Damage

Other types of skin damage are acne, acne scars, or scars of different kinds of injury. These will start fading for you in about two weeks.

Once you start to have daily treatments, you will start seeing a noticeable improvement in four to six weeks. Scientists are continuing to study this type of therapy. At this time, they are encouraged by the results that people are getting, and you can get also

The Seven Main Benefits of Red Light Therapy

When you first hear about red light therapy, you may think that this sounds like something out of a science fiction movie, but Red Light Therapy is a real technique that delivers wavelengths into your skin safely.

With all the rumors toasting it being able to cure everything, here is information that will tell you the real gains for using Red Light Therapy. NBA, Olympians, natural health leaders, gymnasts have all reaped the benefit of red light therapy.

Using Red Light Therapy, means you're going through a safe procedure that involves wavelength of natural light soaking into your skin and right to your cells. Usually, you're either standing or sitting for about 15 minutes a day during the procedure. Your cells drink in the natural light, so the more area it covers, the better off your body will gain from the therapy.

There are many types of devices out there that use Red Light Therapy. For instance, joov delivers quality devices that focus on wave light. Studies in the field of photo medicine looked at the amount of red light and infrared that is the best for your health.

The cells in our bodies take that light and other resources and change it into energy we need. This procedure induces stimulation to collagen, elastin, and fibroblast, which brings about something called ATP, the bringer of energy to every cell in our bodies. Red

Light Therapy facilitates the further growth of ATP.

Many people use Red Light Therapy for the following:

- Skin Care

- Pain Relief

- Revive the Skin

- Improve Eyesight

- Help the Brain

- Clear Acne

- Improve Sleep

Lose Weight

Quite a few experts hold to the belief that Red Light Therapy will help solve skin problems, including scarring, wrinkles, and age spots. When Red Light Therapy targets your cells, it brings about a regenerative factor into the equation, which leaves you with younger-looking skin, a decrease of scars. Red Light Therapy can't make miracles, and if you're considering using the treatment, it should only be one of the steps in your overall plan to improve your skin health.

Evidence does show that this procedure works and is becoming widely available, including going to a spa, dermatologist, or maybe your local gym. You could also do it at home using a Red Light Therapy bed or a red light face mask. If you have the cash, you can buy a red light therapy bed for around 3,000.

Beware that if you decide to go with using a device, make sure you know how much output the device puts out. Some Red Light Therapy devices can be found on Amazon and used in the mornings as well as nights to promote collagen, and they come with remote control. Nowadays, you can even get the treatment through your computer or phone.

However, you are not just using any old red light. For this procedure to work at it best, you must have two wavelengths of redlight that include 660 nanometers and 850 nanometers. The reason why is because 660 nanometer has more available access to permeating your skin. 850 goes even deeper allowing more benefit to your muscle, joint pain, and other parts of your body. Remember to exercise caution at those facilities that change UV bulbs to red bulbs. A trip to a professional means you get a treatment that takes full advantage of the wavelengths.

The Benefits of Using Red Light Therapy

Revive the skin and help with acne. Are you tired of looking your age or older? Studies have shown that Red Light Therapy can help increase collagen in your skin and improve the overall smoothness along with texture, tone, and wrinkles. Plus, your skin will feel more hydrated. Your body is made up of collagen. As you age, your skin loses elasticity because of elastosis. When this happens, you begin to show signs of aging, such as wrinkles.

Quite a few people have benefited from Red Light Therapy treatment because it regenerates cellular function and helps stimulate the production of collagen. There is some evidence that it can help clear up your skin. Red Light Therapy is safe for all types of skin and has been known to diminish acne scarring by getting deep into your skin layer, repairing tissue while also soothing the skin. Red Light Therapy especially works well with a chronic skin condition.

Red Light Therapy can be used either by itself or with blue light therapy. With a plethora of skin cream out there, you may find Red Light Therapy more satisfying.

Pain relief. Another benefit of Red Light Therapy is a decrease in pain. Studies further show that Red Light Therapy stimulates the mitochondrial. It also reduces inflammation. Because of the many research and hundreds of clinical tests done in thirty years using this technique, it has been found that Red Light Therapy has reduced osteoarthritis, knee pain, meniscus tear, rheumatoid arthritis, diabetic foot ulcers, morning stiffness. The evidence is so strong that the FDA has approved Red Light Therapy. In 2018 Brazil's researchers found evidence that Red Light Therapy diminished cytokine levels and promoted the growth of immune cells in mammals.

Sleep improvement. You may have had trouble falling asleep, and perhaps you take supplements in the form of melatonin, but did you know that using Red Light Therapy could improve the quality of sleep you get? Depending on how much artificial light your body comes in contact with, it may take a while before the urge to sleep overcomes you. By using a Red Light Therapy device during the day, clinical tests have provided evidence that it encourages melatonin production in your body, which allows you to get some rest quicker.

Fatigue. Need more energy? Red Light Therapy could give you the boost you need. The ATP harness from Red Light Therapy elevates your body into better performance with more power, which allows you to perform in a variety of physical activities. The evidence has been backed up with many clinical trials, including pro-athletes and weight trainers, who use Red Light Therapy devices to give them a better edge when performing and have a quicker recovery speed.

Improve your eyesight. There have been studies demonstrating that Red Light Therapy decreases macular degeneration of the eyes while increasing your cells' ability to do its job. Red Light Therapy works well with the mitochondria, and since your eyes have an excellent source of mitochondria, it benefits your visit.Increase your circulation and aids the brain. Even more, studies have proven that after Red Light Therapy, circulation increases as more oxygen and nutrients are getting to your tissue. This type of therapy also gives aid in protecting red blood cells against oxidative strives while decreasing platelet loss during a surgical procedure. Help the brain. Research has proven that Red Light Therapy can help those with traumatic injuries to their brain. The therapy is directed toward the head to not only preserve brain cells but regenerative them

Help you lose weight. Those who have researcher Red Light Therapy believe in its effect on adipocytes cells, which store fat. Red Light Therapy assists the body in flushing away fat cells. Furthermore, according to the International Journal of Endocrinology 2012 study, light affects your level of hunger. In an earlier study, tests were done with women in the age category from 25 to 55 and into two groups. One group participates in using a treadmill that includes Red Light Therapy, and the other group performs only with the treadmill.

Scientists who worked on thermographic photographs which highlighted the changes in cellulite with the group that uses both Red Light Therapy and treadmill. The studies found that the first group using Red Light Therapy improved more in their bodies.

Side effects of taking Red Light Therapy are practically nonexistent. Because its origin is natural, it doesn't harm the skin. Red Light Therapy continues to be tested through many clinical trials, and so far, all of them have had positive feedback.

Many studies have been done with Red Light Therapy and with most of them coming from animals. The results have been promising, but the verdict on Red Light Therapy benefits are still linked to controversy. However, the evidence seems to support that it does help.

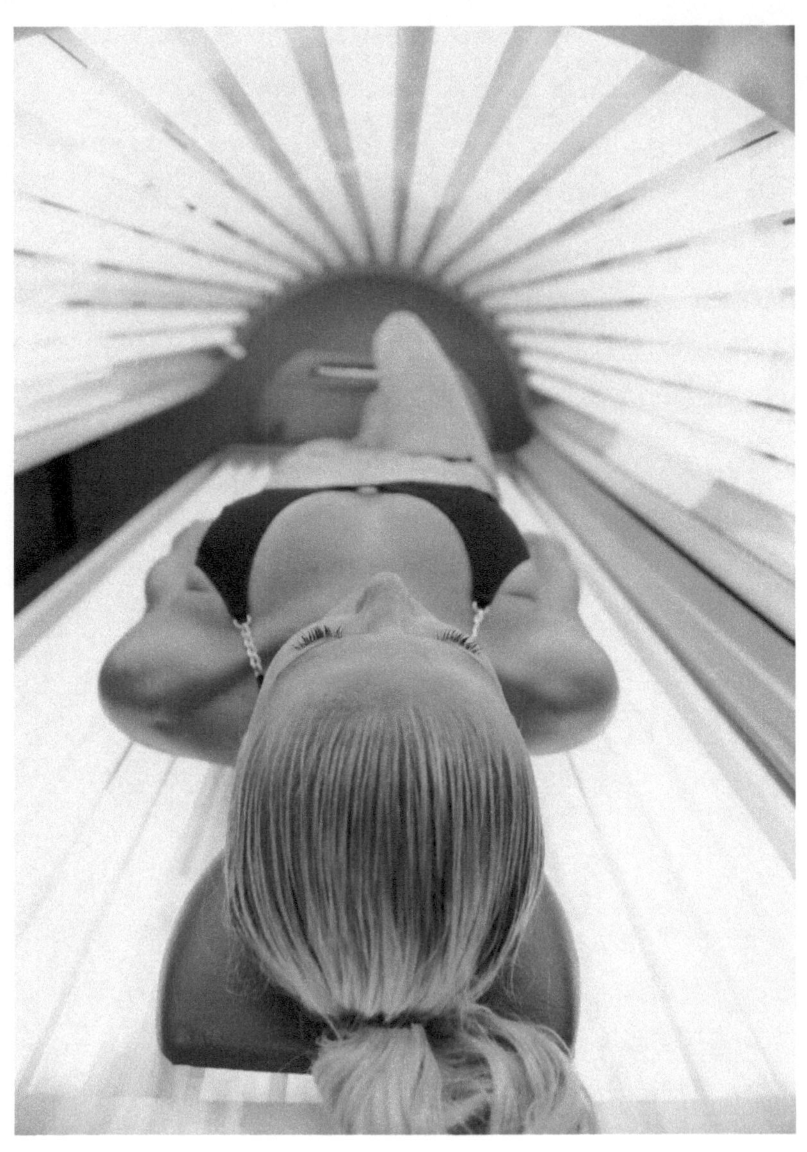

The Best and Worst of Red Light Therapy

Red Light Therapy has become something of a phenomenon recently thanks to the growing community of biohackers across the United States. This therapy, which has been used for the last several decades in salons to help women prevent wrinkles, acne, and dermatological conditions, is said to prompt cellular stimulation, increase the energy of cells, and improve blood flow. First developed by scientists in the 90's as a means to grow plants in space, this "therapy" consists of exposing as much of your skin to red lights that mimic the sun without UV rays.

If you are interested in learning more about red lights or considering buying yourself a lamp, this article is for you. Outlined below are the pros and cons of Red Light Therapy as a technique to complement a healthy lifestyle.

First, some pros!

The reason red lights are rising in popularity is because people who have experimented with them are seeing results. Looking at the sheer length of the list of pros below is likely to create some skepticism. "Some lights can do all that?" The answer is yes. Remember that the founding claim of this red light trend is that these lights increase blood flow, stimulate cell growth, and improve their function. High school biology taught us that the entire body is made up of cells, which implies that improving cell function would improve virtually every other mechanism of the body. Hence the long list. Let's dig into some of these pros.

Stimulates Collagen Production

Collagen is the most abundant protein in our bodies. It can be found in joints, bones, ligaments, muscles -- everywhere. However, our body always needs more of it, especially if we are active or aging. Many people find this additional collagen through supplements, but red lights can help here by stimulating the growth of collagen. When your body produces more collagen, you will notice a difference in the creeks and cracks. Every day, things sometimes trigger. And the difference will be their absence. More collagen equals better, smoother, healthier movement of joints.

Strengthens Immune System

Red lights claim to stimulate cell growth, and healthy cells are precisely what the body needs to fight diseases and infections.

Fights Acne

Acne is an infection of the skin. When the skin cells are more durable and healthier, perhaps thanks to red lights, they will be less susceptible to acne.

Speeds Up Recovery from Injury

Without sounding like a broken record, when we suffer an injury, it is our cells that have to repair and rebuild. Red lights speed up that process.

Heals Wounds and Scars

Same as above, substitute "injury" for "wound" or "scar."

Nourishes Sensitive Skin

Dry skin? Eczema? Redness? All cellular issues, all aided by the healing properties of red lights.

Help with Joint Stiffness and Rheumatoid Arthritis

This is related to number 1, and 4. Where heating pads heat the internal tissues and trigger joint responses by using external heat, red lights activate internal temperature. This therapy offers the same powers as a heating pad, but with less of a daily time commitment and without giving any sensation of heat that you can feel.

Supports Thyroid Function and Healing from other Hormone Issues

Low energy levels, thyroid problems, and hormonal issues are all too familiar in modern America. Red lights address these problems the same way they treat any other, through cellular support.

Reduces Muscle Spasms and Restless Legs

Like so many of the above points, when cells are supported, and collagen is being produced at accelerated rates, bodily aches and pains are greatly minimized, if not altogether absent.

Eases Pain

Related to 7, 4, 9, and 1, this can happen with red lights because of the way the light rays trigger a cellular response.

So what are the cons?

At first, users may have a few concerns about the lights and their eyes and skin. More than one of the points in the "pro" list suggests that red lights are perfect for your skin, so that concern is eliminated. As for your eyes, well, eyes are made of cells (like every other part of your body), and the principal benefit of red lights is supporting cell growth. There isn't much about red lights except for these two things, which impact every choice humans make in the twenty-first century.

Time

To see results, you need to be entirely consistent in your use of the therapy. It takes as little as ten minutes a day for a week to start seeing results, and it is best to continue using the lights at a regular interval. For busy parents or business executives, finding time can be difficult.

Money

Red lights can be as cheap as $20 (for handheld flashlight options) to $250 for at-home kits depending on size and quality. The alternative is going to a gym or spa for treatments which can run from $20-$85 a session.

These cons are nothing compared to the potential benefits using red lights can bring to your life.

Ok, how would I use them?

The trick with red lights is to let as much of your skin be exposed to the rays as possible while standing within four to six inches of them. If there is a specific sore spot or scar you are hoping to heal, then logic follows to place that spot in the center of the light to receive the most of the rays. The length of sessions ranges from as quick as ten minutes to as long as twenty, not longer.

Where can I find them?

As a result of their growing popularity, it is becoming more accessible and easier to find this treatment. There are a variety of companies selling red lights to do the therapy in the comfort of your home. For those uninterested or unable to create a red light space in their house, gyms, spas, and salons, with growing frequency, are investing in these red lights as the demand for the therapy grows. Simply googling the treatment in your area should connect you with someplace close.

Guide to Home Use Red Light Therapy

There is no dispute that our bodies need regular sunlight to maintain optimum health. Our skin soaks up the sun's rays, absorbing the energy it needs to produce a variety of critical vitamins that we use daily.

The most important of these is Vitamin D. The body uses Vitamin D to stimulate brain function, fight inflammation, reduce blood pressure, and improve muscle development. Low Vitamin D levels can weaken the body and even lead to dementia or depression.

However, getting the requisite amount of sunlight every single day can be harder than it sounds. Some people live in areas of inhospitable climate, while others have to contend with a heavy work schedule. Thankfully, if you're one of those, there are still some alternatives available.

Red Light Therapy, for example, is a trend that's gaining popularity. The process uses synthetically generated red or near-infrared light to bolster a variety of bodily systems. Regularly exposing your body to red light can help prevent or alleviate a number of health issues. This includes things like chronic pain, hair loss, inflammation, and weight gain.

It may also have an effect on mental conditions such as fatigue or depression. Officially known as Photobiomodulation, the goal of Red Light Therapy is to use an infrared or near-infrared LED device to energize cells. This, in turn, triggers beneficial chemical reactions throughout the body, increasing health and wellness overall.

These devices are relatively cheap and easy to install—no need to worry about retrofitting a room with solar panels and mucking up the property taxes.

The specific effects of Red Light Therapy depend on the device used. Different devices generate different wavelengths and have different power densities. As such, you'll need to make a careful appraisal of all available options. Which model is the best can be a subject of dispute among users, so consider your personal needs above all else.

Generally speaking, smaller devices only put out enough to bathe the outer skin layer. This is useful for reducing wrinkles and fighting inflammation. However, the lower surface area covered means that therapy sessions will take longer if you want to achieve full-body benefits.

In contrast, larger devices cover more surface area. This not only decreases the length of each therapy session but allows more energy to be absorbed by the skin. Thus, large light panels lack the mobility of a hand-held device but are more useful overall.

A key factor when choosing the best device for your needs is power density. This indicates the intensity of the light. Lights with low power density will not penetrate as far into the skin layer, significantly reducing the benefit of the treatment.

The power density is generally not listed anywhere directly on the device. Instead, it must be extrapolated based on the device's wattage and maximum treatment area. Power Density comes in the form of the equation mW/cm2. An ideal density for full effectiveness is 30mW/cm2, with a range of about six feet.

With the light of appropriate range and power, your daily therapy session should only take a couple of minutes. This means you can get everything you need from a short session and then return to your property taxes. As an added benefit, most devices are highly energy-efficient and will produce minimum strain on your electric bill.

Red Light Therapy is non-invasive, meaning there are limited risks involved. The light's intensity is not enough to require goggles, though color perception may be skewed temporarily after each session. Oversaturation will not result in sunburns as sunlight does, and most devices do not generate heat.

The most significant risk involved is oversaturation, which can limit the overall effectiveness of the treatment but will not cause physical harm.

With a little research and a small daily time investment, you can use Photobiomodulation to strengthen and support your body's natural processes, leading to greater potential health.

Conclusion

In the end, none of this can be handed off as medical fact because, as this article from Harvard states, much of the research is still ongoing and inconclusive. Red Light Therapy is another way that human beings have devised to help achieve their goals in getting their bodies into the best shape and keeping them there. However, given the information above, it seems like the possible advantages make giving the therapy a try a worthy endeavor.

URL: https://www.health.harvard.edu/staying-healthy/led-lights-are-they-a-cure-for-your-skin-woes

Thank You

RLT2020